Stuttering: Power Over It

A liberating and empowering self-help program

Dale F. Williams, Ph.D.

Published by The Brainary® Australia and The Brainary® LLC United States of America.

Registered Office: PO Box 1318, Geelong, Victoria, 3220, Australia

www.thebrainary.com

info@thebrainary.com

First Published by The Brainary May 18 2020

ISBN: 978-0-9873476-5-7 (pbk)

ISBN: 978-0-9873476-6-4 (ebook)

Title: Stuttering: Power Over It: A Liberating and Empowering Self-Help Program©

Author: Dale F. Williams Ph.D.

Illustrations: The Gordon TAFE Geelong 3220 Australia

Marketing support: Deakin University, Australia

The publication is a workbook developed for adults who stutter (or stammer). This workbook is not a replacement for professional treatment by a speech-language pathologist and should not be viewed as a substitute for all that treatment can offer. In fact, it is best used in conjunction with treatment. Additionally, if you are experiencing psychological symptoms or problems in your life, you should seek the help of an experienced mental health professional.

Target Audience: Adults who stutter (or stammer)

Subjects: Stuttering, Speech Disorders, Speech-language pathology

About The Author

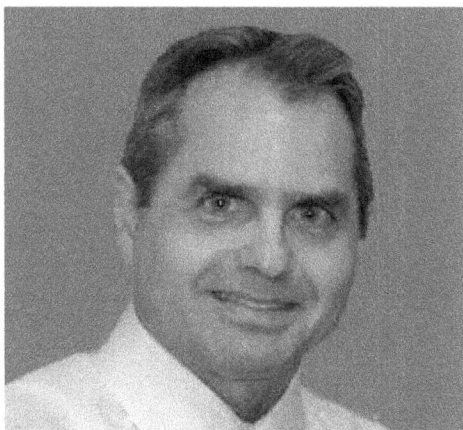

Dale F. Williams, Ph.D., CCC-SLP, BCS-F is Professor and Chair of the Department of Communication Sciences and Disorders at Florida Atlantic University. In addition, he is a consultant for Language Learning Intervention and Professional Speech Services. Dr. Williams completed his bachelor's degree at Alma College, his master's at the University of Oklahoma Health Science Center, and his doctorate at Southern Illinois University. A Board Certified Specialist in Fluency since 1999, Dr. Williams served as Chair of the Specialty Board on Fluency Disorders for three years. His publications are primarily in the area of fluency disorders and include three books (available at https://hearsayresources.com/). A person who stutters, Dr. Williams coordinated the stuttering support group that has met on the FAU campus since 1996. He lives with his wife Misty in Lake Worth Beach, FL, USA, where they raised four children and a wide variety of spoiled pets.

Other Titles by Dale F. Williams, PhD:

- Shining a Light on Stuttering : How One Man Used Comedy to Turn His Impairment Into Applause
- Communication Sciences and Disorders: An Introduction to the Professions
- Stuttering Recovery: Personal and Empirical Perspectives

Available at www.hearsayresources.com

Dedication

To Dale L. Williams, M.D.:
Dad, you may have left us,
but your inspiration lives on.

Acknowledgements

I start with Lindsay Lowy, graduate assistant extraordinaire. For this project, she served as researcher, idea person, and proofreader. Unfortunately, her education took her off campus, where she agreed to help further as a volunteer. All told, her commitment to this project was unfailing.

Losing Lindsay was a setback to be sure. The silver lining turned out to be her replacement, Jillian Scott. When we decided to add a final chapter of stuttering resources, Jillian was up to the task, researching and organizing numerous worldwide resources. I thank her for her dedication and hard work. Same goes for graduate assistant Samantha Gumula, who helped with the final touches.

Of course, every book needs a publisher and The Brainary's Hugh Kingsley filled that role admirably. Our discussions about content, organization, and overall message were among the highlights of the process. I also appreciated his openness to new ideas. When I sent the first draft, I told him only that it was unconventional, making no mention of the science fiction aspects of the story. His response: "I like it." And off we went.

This project did require much work at home, particularly during the coronavirus pandemic, so I appreciate the patience of my family during the completion phase. On the subject of family, I am sad to report that I lost my father during the final editing process. Frankly, I do not know whether he would have liked the story. He was a man of science, but not so much science fiction, preferring spy novels and Westerns.

I thank all people who stutter for their inspiration. In particular, I should recognize those whose stories inspired this book. Your courage in the face of everyday barriers is remarkable.

Having students contribute is not new to me. But having The Gordon TAFE students in Geelong, Australia develop the front cover artwork was rather special. A big thanks to The Gordon TAFE students.

Finally, listeners serve a role as well. Without their understanding, patience, and willingness to learn, there could be no stories. And, yes, I recognize that also holds true for those listeners who lack any of those traits, the ones who ignored, interrupted, sneered, and bullied. They are just harder to thank.

Table of Contents

Note to Readers

This story represents a crossing from identification to acceptance, a journey of personal growth designed to liberate oneself from the bounds of stuttering. Presented here is a means of confronting stuttering and letting go of feelings that have held you back. Many have been controlled far too long by this mysterious condition and are looking for a way to turn the tables and live a full life. This workbook is here to help.

If you're a person who stutters, it is hoped that the journey within these pages can help you find a sense of confidence and security about your speech, to be able to say what you want to say when you want to say it, even if you sometimes stutter. Your thoughts are as important as anyone else's and, therefore, need to be heard.

If you're a speech-language pathologist, I hope this story can provide you with a resource to help navigate those tricky emotional and attitudinal aspects of treatment. I have a mental image of therapists assigning clients a chapter or two at a time for discussion during a later session. Of course, you know your clients and I don't, so any differences you make to that plan are undoubtedly the correct ones.

Regardless of your role in the process, I hope you enjoy the story of an ordinary man and an unwanted companion you will all recognize.

Prologue

What if you could relive past life events?

Think about going back to the first time you met your significant other. Or that time you scored the winning goal or answered the question that had stumped the class. That vacation that was so much more fun than all the others. The people and places you left behind. When the laughter or applause was all for you.

The stuff of science fiction? Well, yes. However, consider that a current theory of memory storage, backed by research, is that long-term memories are warehoused throughout the brain as groups of neurons programmed to reproduce the original event.

But that's remembering, which is, of course, different than experiencing.

Now suppose that you could metaphorically get inside your own head—not just get there, but snoop around until you found what you were looking for. And what if you had the ability—via, say, meditation, hypnosis, prayer, or lucid dreaming—to fire memory-laden neurons with you right smack in the middle of the detonation, carried along for the ride? In such a hypothetical, you should actually experience the event the same as when it happened while still knowing it is a past memory, right?

Well, no. Probably not. It just seems too simple. My guess is that there is something on that giant electrical grid we call a brain—some forgotten variable, process, or force—that would alter my little theory.

Maybe an unwanted visitor accustomed to ruining every situation it inhabits. Something that is difficult—but not impossible—to control.

Chapter 1: Introduction

An evil force arrived to destroy me. Worse yet, I could do nothing to stop it.

So I waited, hoping against hope that it would simply go away. If not forever, then at least for a day. That's all I ever asked: Just leave me alone for one day.

But it was not to be.

I do not recall how I got to where I was and, frankly, I was less interested in that than I was in the image forming before my eyes. Most would have found it forgettable, but I would have said homely. The face was round and pockmarked, the scalp balding, the posture stooped. If my friends were around, I would have pretended it was not there, although they would have known it was.

The formation knew me on sight. I remained silent, unsurprised. I was apprehensive, but not scared. At that moment, the feeling was more anticipation than fear. And, unfortunately, familiarity.

A giant arm gestured for me to follow. I paused and let the creature go ahead. But then I submitted.

As always.

The path we trudged brought me to my childhood bedroom. I had just woken up, going through, as usual, all the speaking situations I was likely to encounter that day. I could sit alone on the bus to school and in the back of the class for first period Geography. Then came Phys Ed, which was basketball that week, meaning I didn't have to yell out any scores or instructions. Then came Anders' class and...oh no. The ugly one smiled, a nasty, mocking grimace that projected no humor.

As soon as the thought struck my brain, I was there: sixth-grade English class. Mrs. Anders was choosing people to diagram sentences on the board. Around my desk, in which I was now seated (when did that happen?), were faces I had not seen in decades and yet I now knew every name, first and last. I was also aware of the class assignment. I was eleven years old again.

Despite my involvement in the scene before me, I knew to look for the one who had brought me there. But when I spotted the form I quickly looked away. It was, quite simply, hideous—the face was gone, covered by scraggly hair and giant warts. The clothes were ragged, and the body oozed some sort of foul liquid onto the classroom floor.

About then Old Lady Anders (who was probably in her early 30s) chose me to diagram sentence number six from the grammar textbook. I walked to the chalkboard, wrote the sentence and diagram, then tried to explain it.

"The subject is...is...is..."

I heard classmates begin to chuckle. I wanted to respond, but the shame within my eleven-year-old brain did not allow it.

"…um, subject is…"

The subject was dog, a word I could not say to save my life. I thought of synonyms that would work—hound, mutt, pooch—but everyone could see that sentence 6 specifically said dog, so word substitution was not a viable option. I looked at the teacher, who just stared at me with a blank expression. I pressed on.

"…duh, duh, duh…" The word was partway out, but the rest was not coming anytime soon. I began to perspire as the laughter grew.

"I don't know what the subject is!" I blurted out. The laughter then reached a roar, as everyone in the room saw through my lie. Even Old Lady Anders was grinning. Until she told me to sit down, that is.

I started the walk of shame back to my seat, but the desk was gone. A breeze hit my face and I knew that I was outside. I was wearing glasses, so I had clearly aged at least a couple years, although I did not really feel any different. I glanced at my companion, who was, if anything, darker and even more hideous than before. The evil grin, however, remained.

Returning my gaze to the scene before me, I immediately saw Duke Nugent blocking my path. Duke was a bully who would torment classmates for another couple of years, until he was old enough to drop out of school and get a job at the local metal casting factory.

"Dude!" he yelled at me. "Wuh-wuh-wuh-wuh-where ya goin'?" Then he laughed at his own alleged cleverness.

Duke was wearing jeans with holes in both knees and a dirty shirt with the logo of some long forgotten heavy metal band. I was afraid to look down at my own clothing, for fear I looked equally ridiculous.

Apparently, I became lost in matters of fashion too long because Duke said, "You checkin' me out Pee-Wee?"

"Nnnnnno," I heard myself say. What was that all about? I wondered. I don't remember ever stuttering on /n/'s before.

"I say—sorry, sssssssay—you are!" he answered.

I looked at Duke's face. The years had erased how terrifying he had always appeared to me. My young brain offered no words of response.

"Yeah, you better keep your mouth shut, Pee-Wee," he said, pushing me out of the way and joining some friends who had evidently witnessed our encounter.

What was happening? I'm a grown man—granted, one stuck in a middle school body—but an adult in real life. Why was I letting some overgrown tweener push me around?

I was angry, mostly at myself for saying nothing. But my anger quickly found another target.

Unsightly or not, my new companion was going to hear from me.

"Why are you doing this?" I asked.

There was no response.

"Do I have to relive all my life's humiliations? What comes next—I bomb out meeting women, public speaking, and saying my own name?"

After another pause, I heard, "Let me show you something."

Before I could protest that I had been shown quite enough already, the creature transformed into something sort of like a humanoid biker movie villain. The hair was long and greasy, the features sharp, and the smell atrocious, though at least it no longer oozed. For my part, I was at a counter, ordering pizza. I had my wallet out, so I must have been an adult.

"Whaddaya want on your slice?" asked the young man behind the counter. Tall and muscular, he spoke with a pattern that was quick and demanding. He was clearly someone accustomed to intimidating others.

What I wanted was pepperoni and as soon as I realized that, I knew I would be unable to say it. Still, I wanted to try.

"Peh-peh-peh-peh-"

"Come on," said Muscles, "Spuh-spuh-spit it out."

I stopped. "Did you just make fun of my stuttering, you @#$%!* &*%#@ @!#*^?!"

(Wow, I had a foul mouth in those days.)

My listener was surprised and did not answer.

"Geh-get the manager," I said.

"Hey, it's cool man. I'm sorry. Tell you what—I'll pay for your slice."

I considered that while he pleaded with his eyes.

"Yeah, OK," I finally said.

I grabbed the pizza and turned around. My companion was there.

"Revenge is sweet."

"Yeah, great," I answered. "And my reward is a piece of pizza that's barely warm and that Musclehead probably spit on."

"He didn't. But what I meant was revenge for Duke Nugent."

"There's a little problem with that. The pizza guy wasn't Duke Nugent. Totally different person."

My companion shrugged. "Not to me."

Questions:

The companion is part of every scenario, yet only the narrator seems to know he's there. Can you explain that?

_____

_____

_____

_____

_____

_____

_____

For most of the chapter, the narrator is a middle-schooler. How would you have portrayed your stuttering at that age? Write a description or draw a picture of your stuttering as you viewed it when you were in middle school.

_____

_____

_____

_____

_____

What other matters made you self-conscious at that age? Were those more, less, or the same as stuttering in terms of anxiety?

_____

_____

_____

_____

_____

_____

_____

The narrator experiences or mentions numerous words and situations that he fears because of his stuttering. Make a list of your own word and situational fears.

People who stutter present secondary behaviors and, for most, it's a long list. The narrator wanted to substitute another word for "dog" and, later, retreated from possible verbal confrontation. What sorts of behaviors have you used to escape or avoid stuttering?

Stuttering brought the narrator feelings of anxiety, shame, embarrassment, self-doubt, guilt, anger, and fear, among others. What emotions have you experienced as a result of stuttering?

What is your version of the narrator's experience in Old Lady Anders' class?

_____

_____

_____

_____

_____

_____

What is your version of the encounter with Duke Nugent? How about the one with the pizza guy?

_____

_____

_____

_____

_____

_____

_____

_____

The narrator is forced to recall how frightened he was of Duke. He also feels he never evened the score. Why do you think encounters with a middle school bully stayed with him so long?

_____

_____

_____

_____

_____

_____

Were you ever teased or bullied for reasons other than stuttering? How was that different?

Why might the companion view painful memories as positive?

How would standing up to a pizza seller as an adult be revenge against a middle school bully?

Chapter 2: Sounds

Once I left my muscle-bound friend at the pizzeria, things started to move fast. The whirlwind began with me behind the wheel of my old Plymouth Horizon, driving through the midwestern United States. I must have been in my twenties, as that is the only time I ever drove cross-country. My traveling companion was in the passenger seat, looking and smelling as if it had been days since the last shower. I kept my eyes on the road, still unsure where I was traveling. A green exit sign came into view. On it was an arrow and a single destination.

Des Moines.

The name of the city triggered something in my brain. It was a unique combination of sounds that I do not believe I would have been able to say under any circumstances. I looked to my right and my companion was gone. But even alone, I could not start the word.

"D-d-d-"

"Deh-deh-deh-deh-"

It is rare that I stutter when I am by myself, but that word was too much for me. I started to wonder why, then realized that the steering wheel was gone.

I would have panicked, but my new surroundings quickly came into focus. I was still seated, but inside a dark theater. An actor on stage was asked how he felt about seeing his past love again. He paused until the theater was dead quiet, then delivered his line beautifully and to great laughter.

"Bittersweet."

The thought of being onstage and having to project that word in such a key spot placed a flock of butterflies in my stomach. I had just watched someone perform an act at which I would have failed miserably. What would I have done if I were in his place and it was my job to say such a difficult word?

Again, I had little time to ponder, as I became distracted by a horrible smell. My companion was back, but now the time since the last shower was well beyond days. Months, perhaps.

I was in a high school classroom. Six people had moved their desks into a small circle. Obviously, some sort of group project was taking place.

Janice Peters was holding a notecard. I had never particularly liked her in those years. She was loud, brash, and her tone always sounded mocking to me. I put up with her, however, because she was friends with Cyndi VanderRoo, my high school crush.

I looked to Janice's right and saw, of all people, Cyndi VanderRoo. Great. Whatever I did next, I better not stutter.

"Your turn," Janice said to me, then looked down at her card.

"Oh, man! You got the easy one!"

She showed her card to Craig Reynolds, the brain of the history class.

He laughed. "If you don't know this one, I feel sorry for you."

Janice read: "On November 9. 1863, Lincoln gave his famous speech at...?"

Gettysburg, of course. I started to give the answer but could feel the first sound catch in the back of my throat. I knew if I pushed too hard, my face would contort while the sound stayed where it was—on the inside. I did not know what to do.

Janice Peters was grinning. Cyndi VanderRoo was looking at me, which increased the pressure to answer quickly.

"I don't know," I said.

The other five students laughed.

"You're joking, right?" asked Craig Reynolds.

I shook my head, looking away before anyone could see my face flush. But when I gazed back, the classroom was empty, save for me and my companion.

"Man, I hate you," I said.

"Plosives are sounds in which the vocal tract is momentarily blocked, then the air is released all at once."

"Thank you, Webster's."

My comment was ignored. "Specifically, plosive sounds are b, p, d, t, g, and k."

Each one of the six cut me like a knife. I despised them all.

Questions:

Go back to your list of feared words from chapter 1. Note any patterns you see.

Have you ever stuttered when alone? Heard a word you would not be able to say in any circumstance? Avoided a word that was too hard to say? Write an anecdote that is your version of having to say Des Moines, bittersweet, or Gettysburg.

Why did he not want to stutter in front of Cyndi VanderRoo? If he had, what's likely to have happened?

Why did the companion become more offensive moving from the first scene to the third?

Chapter 3: Situations

My travels across the memory banks finally provided a pleasant surprise: I landed in a small pub, across the table from Bill. He was one of the few friends I made as an adult and it was a friendship that had lasted for decades.

Neither of us were big drinkers. We met in the pub periodically to catch up because it was halfway between our houses.

I was always surprised that Bill made time for me, as he was one of those guys who always seemed to be in a hurry.

As the scene came into focus, there was more good news: My time travel companion was nowhere to be found.

"How's work?" Bill was asking when I arrived.

Somehow, I knew how exactly to respond. "It's all right, though I get tired of—"

"Co-workers? Me too. Just something we all have to put up with. There's this one guy—"

"I was going to say—"

"What?"

Out of the corner of my eye, I spotted my companion, looking like just another ugly guy in a bar. I could feel my jaw start to tense. I looked back at Bill. "I wasn't talking about—"

"Not co-workers? What then?"

"I get tuh-tuh-tuh—"

"Tired, yeah, I got that. Tired of what?"

I sighed, an unsuccessful attempt to relax my mouth. "Office puh—"

"Politics? Ain't that the truth? There's this one guy…" and off he went on a story. I never did get to hear what "this one guy" did however, because Bill's voice was replaced by that of a man in a suit, seated behind an office desk. Behind him stood my companion, looking basically like he had in the pub, albeit dirtier.

"Tell me about yourself," the seated man instructed.

Ah, a job interview. I did not recognize the guy, so apparently it was for a job I did not get.

"Well, I'm looking for an entry level puh—, um, job. Uh, any duh-de-, um 'epartment would be fine though I prefer sssssssome over, you know, others."

The interviewer gave me a puzzled look and I could feel my blood pressure rise. We sat in silence for what was probably only a few seconds, but still seemed too long. Then I watched the interviewer's face lengthen and darken. The result was weird: He had morphed into comedian Elliott Weiss. I was a fan and had met Mr. Weiss when he performed at my college. It was a coincidental meeting in the university theater men's room.

That's where I found myself again, just Elliott Weiss, me, and, probably hiding nearby, the monster.

I was washing my hands and staring at the comedian, my brain momentarily paralyzed by the incongruity of seeing a television personality in real life.

He nodded at me.

"Hi," I managed.

He stuck out his hand and said, "Elliott Weiss."

My hands were still wet, but I did not consider that. I just grabbed his outstretched palm and started to introduce myself. My name was difficult to say under ordinary circumstances. In this situation, I could tell as soon as I opened my mouth that the word had no intention of leaving my throat. All I felt were several long seconds of tension. Elliott Weiss patiently waited—or at least I think he did as I dropped eye contact during my struggle.

Just before I would have choked from lack of breathing, my name finally popped free.

"Nice to meet you," he said, and exited the bathroom with a friendly smile.

When it originally happened, the embarrassment of that meeting had stayed with me for weeks. This time, however, I could not dwell on it. My companion again had me on the move.

The next voice I heard was that of my brother Aaron. He and I were seated at the family dinner table along with Mom and Dad. My companion was also there, and dressed for dinner.

"Who smells?" asked Aaron.

"Don't start with that," warned Mom.

"All right then, who doesn't smell, you know, pleasant?" asked my dad. Often, Dad was as silly as his kids, so Mom was outnumbered.

"I don't know whether to raise my hand or not," I said quickly.

As soon as I finished, Dad said, "Only if you smell."

"Dear! Really!"

"A better question is why does someone smell," said Aaron.

"Or maybe why doesn't someone smell, you know, pleasant."

"No one smells," argued Mom. "Change the subject."

"Theh-theh-then change something else," I offered.

"Such as?"

"Habits, hygiene, cuh-cuh-cuh-cleanliness."

"Underwear," suggested Dad.

"Yeah, that too."

Someone started laughing, but I was drifting away. When I stopped, I was seated at a different dining table, this one in my college cafeteria. Everyone at the table was my friend. The one speaking was looking directly at me.

"I agree," he said. "A single-elimination tournament is the dumbest way possible to pick a college basketball champion." There was a brief pause before someone from across the table spoke.

"What do you want them to do, play four of seven like the NBA?" he asked. "You can't have college kids playing into June."

"Single-elimination isn't valid," I argued. "Too high a random factor. Play the tournament twice and   you'd get four different teams in the final four."

Everyone was eating, so another pause followed.

"Some years that's true," my college roommate agreed between bites. "But sometimes one team is dominant. Besides, the NBA sucks."

I thought about that. "The NBA's suckery has nothing to do with the issue at hand. Theirs is a more valid way to decide a champion." With that I took a bite of my burger.

"Hmm…you know, actually, it is relevant. The college game is more exciting because of single elimination!"

I finished chewing, then responded. "Exciting, maybe. But when it's over, we don't really know who the best team is."

Someone who had not yet chimed in gestured for attention as he swallowed a bite. When we looked his way, he spoke.

"Yes, we do, if we define best as team that wins the tourney."

I started to say something about the how if we don't care about randomness, we should stop playing the tournament and just draw a team name out of a hat, but I had to squint at bright lights that were suddenly in my eyes. I looked down to see that I was dressed in a suit and standing behind a podium. I knew immediately that I was delivering a speech on the topic of my stuttering and what my next thought was.

"Learning that stuttering has a neurological buh-um, I mean, basis was empowering to me, because that was when I understood that it was not my fault."

A hand shot up amongst the few people in the audience. "I know a guy who told his kid he better not hear any more stuttering and the kid stopped. Doesn't sound neurological to me."

I smiled. This one was too easy.

"Recovery does happen with children, often spontaneously. When it does, there's a tendency to associate unrelated events with the recovery."

My questioner nodded, then morphed into Ray, a co-worker I had always liked. We were in a meeting and, I quickly realized, I was running it.

"If the hours stay the same, how do we save money?" Ray was asking me.

"We don't," I answered, "unless we increase the hours enough over four days that we can keep the building closed on Fridays."

"Would we have access to it on Fridays?" asked Paul, another subordinate.

"Yes, but not the thermostat. That's how they're saving money. It'll probably feel too cold on winter Fridays and too hot in the summer."

"You sure have all the answers," said another attendee I did not recognize at first. I stared at him until I noticed that he and I were the only ones left in the conference room.

"It's me," said my companion. "You didn't notice me in the cafeteria or during your speech either."

"Sometimes you just blend in," I admitted.

Questions:

With sounds, patterns may be clear—such as difficulty with plosives. But what is the pattern with the narrator's difficult and easy speaking situations?

_____

_____

_____

_____

_____

Look at your list of difficult situations from chapter 1 and write down any patterns you see, be they external (for example, certain people or personalities that are difficult to deal with) or internal (the way they make you feel or otherwise affect you)?

_____

_____

_____

_____

_____

_____

Why was the companion missing when the narrator first met his friend Bill?

_____

_____

_____

Why was it dressed for dinner with the family?

_____

_____

_____

Why does it blend into some situations?

Was the narrator relatively comfortable in situations in which he gave himself permission to stutter? Why might that be important?

The most difficult situations were talking to Bill the interrupter, interviewing for a job, and saying his own name. The easiest were talking to friends, giving a speech about stuttering, and running a meeting. Talking with family fell in the middle—the speaker was relaxed but disfluent. Would the relative difficulty of these situations be the same for you? If not, how would they differ?

Why did he lose eye contact when struggling with his name? Have you ever done that? Would it be better or worse to maintain eye contact in that situation? Explain your answer.

_____

_____

_____

_____

_____

_____

Is speaking with family an easy or difficult situation for you? Why?

_____

_____

_____

_____

_____

_____

_____

Why do you think talking about basketball with friends was easy for the speaker?

_____

_____

_____

_____

_____

_____

_____

_____

When looking for patterns, did you write down the word stress or pressure? If so, define it.

Describe in writing a difficult speaking situation you experienced. Then an easy one.

What did you feel as you wrote these descriptions? What did you learn?

Chapter 4: Name that emotion

"Let's review," my companion continued. "I'll name a place we visited, you tell me how you felt."

I sighed. "Fine."

"Des Moines road sign."

"Anxious."

"The 'bittersweet' moment in the play."

"Nervous."

"History class discussing Gettysburg."

"Shame, humiliation."

"Job interview."

"Annoyance, then weakness."

"Meeting Elliott Weiss."

"Embarrassment."

"Don't you ever feel any positive emotions?"

"Keep going," I said.

"Family dinner."

"Comfortable."

"But you were stuttering."

"Comfortable."

"Arguing basketball in college."

"Accepted."

"Giving a speech."

"Confident."

"Why?"

I had to think about that one. "I guess because it was about stuttering."

Questions:

How would you have felt in each of the situations described?

_____

_____

_____

_____

_____

_____

_____

_____

Give examples of occasions in which you experienced anxiety, nervousness, humiliation, shame, annoyance, weakness, and embarrassment.

_____

_____

_____

_____

_____

_____

_____

_____

Give examples of occasions in which you experienced comfort, acceptance, and confidence.

_____

_____

_____

_____

_____

_____

_____

_____

What are the differences between the two sets of examples above (that is, how do the two sets of situations differ)?

Public speaking is normally difficult. Why might giving a speech about stuttering be associated with positive emotion?

Read the following quote:

The problems with taking risks in such feared circumstances are 1) by definition, they sometimes go wrong, leaving the risk-taker with a sense of loss, and 2) individuals tend to overestimate the probability of failed risks...Perhaps because of these reasons, people are generally risk averse...Exceptions to this aversion seem to occur in instances in which we have given ourselves permission to fail...It's easy to take risks when the cost of failure is nothing more than a moment of awkwardness one can easily move past. However, such is not the case when, say, a speaker has no idea how new listeners are going to respond when surprised by a speech difference. In that scenario, the fear of failure is pronounced and taking risks can seem exceedingly difficult (Williams & Campbell, 2016).

Does risk-taking apply to any of the situations experienced in this chapter? Does either one apply to you? Why or why not?

Chapter 5: Secondary behaviors

I grabbed a chair and sat down at the conference table. Only it wasn't a conference table any longer. It was a therapy desk and I was back in the speech room of my middle school. It was a small space, barely large enough for the desk, chairs, and the three who were present—me, the speech-language pathologist, and an unsightly presence that I could now easily recognize as my traveling partner.

"What happens when you try to say your name?" the SLP was asking me.

"I'll show you," said my 13-year-old self. "My name is…"

Immediately I felt my lips and jaw tighten. Then my throat constricted as the muscle tension increased geometrically, keeping the word safely locked inside.

I was going to smack the table to aid in releasing the word, but there was a plastic ashtray in the spot where my palm would have landed. So instead I grabbed the ashtray and threw it down as hard as I could against the polished surface.

The combination of the throwing motion and the clang of object hitting table worked. As my name burst free from the stutter, however, I saw the ashtray bounce off the surface and strike the SLP in the forehead. I started to apologize, but the SLP was now my college roommate and the treatment room the dormitory TV lounge. It was obviously a warm day, as we were both dressed in shorts and t-shirts. Evidently, we were engaged in some sort of philosophical discussion.

"How do you know people's politics aren't in their DNA?" he asked me.

Good question, I thought.

"Fine inquiry," I said.

"Fine inquiry? What does that even mean?"

"It means I thought…um, you know, what you asked was, well, guh—um, not awful."

"Uh huh. Thanks for clarifying. Sure wish you came with subtitles."

He continued. "What do you think about graduate school?"

I noticed I was now wearing a winter sweater and the TV lounge had changed to the dorm room we shared during what—junior year? Senior?

Same listener, different conversation.

"What?" I asked.

"Try to keep up. I said: What do you think about grad school?"

Good question, I thought.

Fine inquiry, I reconsidered.

"Ffffff…" I said.

"You spring a leak? I asked you…"

"Worthy interrogative," I said.

"What?"

I could not think of a response that I could actually say, so I gave him the thumbs up sign. The conversation ended with my roommate rolling his eyes. Except he was no longer my roommate. Instead, I was staring at Mr. Ellis, my sophomore-year high school English teacher. I instinctively understood why eye rolling had brought me to him. He was doing exactly that as I approached his desk.

"Here," he said, handing me the hall pass before I had even asked for it. I was the only student who ever asked to go to the bathroom during class and did so at least three times a week. I am sure Mr. Ellis thought I had the weakest bladder in recorded history.

I grabbed the pass and went into the hallway where I felt safe. Mr. Ellis had announced that he was going to choose students to diagram sentences on the board and then name the subject, verb, object, and all modifiers. He usually chose five or six people for diagraming, so I figured if I stayed out of the classroom for ten minutes, I was safe.

Sure enough, when I returned, all of the students were quietly working at their desks. Nobody was presenting. Crisis averted, I got the assignment from Mr. Ellis and took my seat.

With about fifteen minutes to go in the class, Mr. Ellis announced, "This is a good time to resume diagramming. Cindy, take sentence number six."

As Cindy approached the board, I again walked to the teacher's desk and asked for the hall pass. For good measure, I held my stomach as if I was queasy.

With a sigh, Mr. Ellis handed over the pass and I left. This time I waited until there were only a few minutes left in the class period before returning. I entered the classroom certain that I had beaten the system again.

It was then that I saw my companion grinning. As I processed this development, Mr. Ellis looked at me and said, "Oh good, you're back. We saved the last sentence for you. Diagram sentence ten for us."

Now I really was queasy. Not only did I have to speak to the class, but there was the added embarrassment of knowing that the teacher, and probably everybody else, had been keeping track of how long I was in the bathroom. Plus, I am sure, many had figured out that I was there only because I was afraid of presenting.

Sentence ten read, "The dog jogged across the park toward my office building."

Why did I always get the dog sentences?

I walked to the board and wrote slowly, hoping time would run out before I had to speak. That did not work, so I tried a new strategy.

"The subject is *cough* d-*cough* duh- *cough* *cough* og, the verb is *cough* ogged *cough* *cough*"

It was about then that the rest of the students disappeared, replaced by a group of camp counselors seated in a cabin. It was an orientation for one of the summer jobs

I worked during my college years.

The camp director had charged us with introducing ourselves one-by-one, just name and where we were from. Both of those words started with problem sounds, so basically I was about to embarrass myself royally in front of the boss, my new peer group, and, of course, my smirking companion.

As I awaited my turn, growing progressively anxious with each new introduction, I heard someone named Bob say he was from Owosso, Oklahoma, a town I had once driven through. When he said it, it did not sound like "Oh-WAH-so," my pronunciation when I was there; it was more like "a-WAH-sa." That gave me an idea.

Although I grew up within shouting distance of the Canadian border, I could always do a decent southern accent. Even better, when I did—mostly just goofing off with my friends—I did not stutter.

After a quick internal listing of southern states, I determined I would be from Louisiana, as it seemed like an easy word to say even without the phony accent. I decided to avoid major cities so I wouldn't have to talk about places people might be familiar with. The trouble was that I had never been to Louisiana and thus did not know any small towns in the state. Therefore, I made one up.

"Where's Lake, Louisiana?" someone asked after I had completed my introduction.

"Um…kind of, er, I mean, pert near Nawlins."

"What's it like?"

And so it began. For the next three months, I lived a lie. Among other false highlights, I graduated from Lake High School, home of the fightin' Lakers, but rarely made the trip over to New Orleans, which is why I was so unfamiliar with the city. The reason my accent came and went was probably because I was going to college up north.

The most uncomfortable conversation that summer was when someone surprised me with the news that there really was a Lake, Louisiana and it was an unincorporated area in the eastern half of the state. Asked what government oversaw the schools, restaurants, movie theaters, and everything else I had mentioned about my alleged hometown, I simply pled ignorance. After all, I could not make up another town when talking to someone who had access to a map.

Fortunately, this time I did not have to re-experience the summer of my new identity, as the scene began to change again.

Questions:

Several secondary behaviors—both verbal actions, general motor movements, and even complete avoidance of speaking —were described in this chapter. The narrator substituted words and feigned an accent. He also threw an object and walked out of a classroom. At the end of chapter 2, you made a list of your secondary behaviors. How many are verbal and how many are more general movements? Can you explain the division of your behaviors?

_____

_____

_____

_____

_____

Do you need to add more behaviors to your list? If so, please do so.

_____

_____

_____

_____

_____

Note which behaviors on your list are used to escape moments of stuttering in progress (such as throwing something or coughing) vs. avoiding it altogether (for example, substituting an easier word, faking an accent, or leaving the room)?

_____

_____

_____

_____

Which are the most and least effective secondary behaviors on your list?

What's a notable secondary behavior moment from your past (such as throwing an object that strikes an authority figure)? Did you regret the action?

What are some potential problems with substituting an easier word for one that is about to be stuttered? Have you ever been caught in a situation in which your speech sounded unnatural because of a secondary behavior? If so, describe.

Have you ever completely and/or unnaturally avoided a situation—pretended to be sick to miss a book report, skipping the first day of school because you might have to introduce yourself, or even unnecessarily visiting the bathroom—because of stuttering?

The combination of faking an accent and devising a new persona is quite an elaborate secondary behavior. What is the most complex secondary behavior in which you have engaged? How do you feel about that behavior now?

In each of the situations you noted in the previous answers (memorable, unnatural, and extreme instances of secondary behavior use), what do you think would have happened had you just stuttered?

Look at your updated list of secondary behaviors. Are any of them now habits or would all of them be easy to stop if you had to?

Why do you think speech-language pathologists caution against using secondary behaviors?

Make a list of secondary behaviors you once used but no longer do. Why did you stop using them?

Why do you think "fine inquiry" was once easy for him to say but no longer is?

It is quite common for secondary behaviors to stop working after a time. Have you ever used one repeatedly that stopped working, such as substituting "fine inquiry" for "good question"? Were you frustrated that, by using a secondary behavior, you had turned one difficult word or situation into two (and then three and four, etc.)? Describe your experience.

Why do you think these behaviors lose their effectiveness? What does it say about the value of using these behaviors?

Rather than letting people in on his secret, the narrator preferred to confuse his roommate with unusual phrasing, let his teacher believe he had some sort of bladder issue, and pretended to be from somewhere he had never even been. What does that say about stuttering?

Chapter 6: Reality

I found myself out for a walk on a pleasant spring day. The neighborhood was quiet and an empty sidewalk stretched before me. The otherwise perfect scenario was marred only by my companion. I could not see him, but I knew he was nearby.

Just as I was coming to this realization, a car passed slowly. I watched as brake lights, then reverse lights, activated. The car backed up until it was even with me. The passenger side window came down and the driver leaned toward it.

"Excuse me. Do you know where Churchill Elementary School is?"

I did. It was on Porter, a word I could not utter under any circumstances.

"Go right on Puh-puh-puh… um, right on, well, um, take a right on Puh-puh-puh-puh-porter." The word burst forth loud and distorted. "Go to the end of the road. The school will be right in front of you."

"Porter?"

I felt my face heat as I nodded.

The driver gestured thanks and took off.

"How did that go?" asked my companion. Its form was again human, but ugly. Not monster ugly. More bulldog ugly.

"Demeaning," I answered.

"How so?"

"How so?! As soon as I started struggling, the guh-guh-guy was sorry he had asked. I guh-guess it's good that he had the willpower to wait for the answer, but then he left without another word. Wasn't it obvious I'd made him uncomfortable?"

"Interesting."

I sighed. "What does that mean?"

"I'll tell you what I saw. A man needed directions. He stopped and asked for directions. Someone gave the man directions. The man, no longer in need of directions, went on about his business."

"That's one way of looking at it, I guh- um, I suppose. But it was still embarrassing."

"Why?"

"Because I stuttered."

"Seems like you'd be used to that."

"That's the puh-pruh-problem. There's never a break. I stutter all the time."

"All the time?"

"Every time I talk."

"What would you estimate is the ratio of free-flowing words to broken ones in your speech?"

"Maybe two to one. On good days three."

"Uh huh. What about the members of your family?"

"All their words are free-flowing."

"Friends?"

"Same."

"Co-workers?"

"Same."

Then my companion was gone, replaced by Ray, a colleague making a reappearance in this adventure. As he came into focus, he was leaning against the doorframe of my office. I was seated at my desk.

"Are you a cat person or a dog person?" Ray was asking me.

Ah, goofing off at work time.

"I hate that question," I answered.

"Why?"

"It's like, well, why does everyone have to be one or the other?"

"Ahh...I guess it's like, y'know, heads or tails. Two choices. Just the way it works."

"More like sandwich puh-pruh-preferences."

"Yeah, um...you're going to have to explain that one."

"OK, uhh...see...nobody ever asks, are you a hot dog puh-puh-puh-person or a hamburger person, making you chuh-choo-choose just one, after which you have to spend the rest of your life insulting whichever one you duh-dih-didn't choose."

"Hmm...you might have a point."

I must have had a great point, given that Ray was usually the type to argue nonsense as long as he could to avoid work.

"And," he added, "your ratio of words to breaks was about seven and a half to one."

I looked at him but, of course he was no longer Ray.

"Not awful," I admitted to my nemesis, at that point looking more like a disheveled old man than a monster.

"Ray's was about nine to one. Break the conversation into syllables instead of words and he's only percentage points ahead of you."

I replayed the conversation in my head as best I could.

"OK," I finally said. "The gap between my speech and others' is not as big as I thought—for total breakdowns. But his are 'ah's and 'um's. Nobody even hears those. Mine call attention to themselves."

My argument was dismissed with a wave of a giant hand. My companion disappeared. Apparently, the point had been made.

Questions:

Describe a scenario in which you were embarrassed to stutter. Include your thoughts at the time and the effects on the listeners.

Now take out all of your own perceptions (e.g., "the guy was sorry he had asked, I'd made him uncomfortable") and just list the facts.

Do you believe at least some of your reactions might have been based more on your own perceptions than the facts? Explain.

What would you estimate your ratio of free-flowing words to disfluent ones (or percentage of words stuttered) is? What about the people you talk to on a daily basis?

Record a conversation and keep track of how often your speech breaks down as well as the speech of whomever you're talking to. What did you find out?

At the end of the chapter, the narrator states that, although his speech may not break down any more than anyone else's, the types of breakdowns make his experience more negative. State whether you agree or disagree with that statement and why.

Chapter 7: Speak Up

Our next stop was another conference room. As was typical by that point, I knew exactly why I was there. I was part of an advisory committee, tasked with researching new technologies for local schools. It was the first meeting and, as such, I did not know anybody in the room. Nor would I get to know any of them. This would be our only gathering, after which we would complete our assigned research and correspond via email.

The meeting chair began with those words all stuttering individuals fear. "Since I don't think everybody knows everybody else, let's start by going around the table and having everyone introduce themselves."

As always seems to happen in these situations, he started on the other side of the table, giving me too much time to think about what I had to say.

My choices were three. I could state my name and hope for the best. I could think of a trick to avoid saying my name—give myself a nickname or pass out my business card, something like that. Or I could openly and voluntarily stutter.

As the first few committee members said their names—all of which I immediately forgot—I looked at my companion. It did not look so bad. It didn't look good, mind you, but at least it wasn't repulsive.

As my turn was nearing, I quickly reviewed the situation. Nobody knew me. I would never see any of these people again. And I was about to say something—my name—that nearly always triggered a stutter. It really was a perfect opportunity to be open about stuttering, as there was so little to lose. I was confident that I would do so. It was just a matter of how I would be honest and open.

- I could self-disclose, perhaps with a joke. "I want to say thank you because for people who stutter, introducing ourselves to a group of strangers is what we live for!"

- I could ease my way through the stutter, using an easy stretch or a bounce, as I had learned in therapy. "Mmmmmy name is..." or "M-m-m-m-my name is..."

- Or I could throw strategy out the window and just stutter with all the tension I'm capable of, but do it with no embarrassment or shame, instead presenting an attitude of here's-my-stutter-deal-with-it.

It was nearly my turn. While the person next to me introduced himself, I felt my load of confidence evaporate like blood through a wound. I glanced at my companion, who was noticeably uglier, especially given the mocking smile spread across its face. Suddenly, everybody was looking at me and I had to speak.

"Mmmm—" Thinking quickly, I made a hoarse growling sound as I gently touched my throat. Then I waved one hand while pointing to my voice box with the other. I was determined to sell the idea that I had lost my voice.

Whether they bought the ruse or not, I cannot say, because at that point I held a pen in the air and, when everybody looked at it, I wrote my name in large block letters on a piece of notebook paper.

What I should have written was Fail.

Questions:

The narrator was granted a relatively safe situation in which to be open about his stuttering. And yet he chickened out. Why?

_____

_____

_____

_____

_____

_____

People who stutter need to get desensitized to reactions—listeners' and their own. Why do you think that process is so often easier said than done?

_____

_____

_____

_____

_____

_____

Were you ever in a circumstance in which you wanted to be up front about your stuttering but were not? Write out a situation from your life that most closely approximates that feeling.

_____

_____

_____

_____

_____

_____

The narrator had plenty of time to prepare to speak. Was that good or bad? Explain your answer.

Which of his three options (the bullet points)—or what combination of them—do you believe he should he have used? Why? What would you have done?

Would you ever stutter easily (option 2)? Why or why not?

Was avoiding the feared word worth it? Why or why not?

How does he feel about himself now? Explain.

Look at your list of difficult situations from chapter 1. Take 2 or 3 of the most difficult ones and brainstorm solutions for how to handle them. Don't overthink your list, just write down your ideas as they pop into your brain.

Do any of your solutions involve self-disclosure, open stuttering, or other means of "avoiding avoidance" (that is, preventing yourself from engaging in avoidance behaviors)? Why do you believe one or all of them could be effective?

_____

_____

_____

_____

_____

_____

_____

_____

Which solutions would you rank as the best? Which are the most realistic? Are your answers the same for both?

_____

_____

_____

_____

_____

_____

_____

_____

The next scene was so similar to the one just completed that I barely noticed the change. The meeting room was about the same size and arrangement. However, the participants were different and more familiar.

I was now in a work meeting and the atmosphere was getting lively. Corporate headquarters had a test they wanted us to give all applicants, though they said we could use the results as we saw fit. On that last point, everyone had an opinion to express.

Well, almost everyone.

The test had two parts, labeled Communication and Computation. Both were scored from 0 to 100.

"Our company deals more with communicating than math. We should take higher com scores," was the first suggestion made.

We don't even know what goes into either of those two scores, I thought. How can we possibly decide that one works better based on what it's called?

"That makes sense," said another voice. "Maybe require a 50 in computation but an 80 in communication?"

Nods of agreement followed this idea.

"Seems like too big a gap," argued a woman on my side of the table. "Maybe 60 and 70."

"Let's split the difference," offered someone new. "Go with 55 and 75."

Why do we need minimums for both parts?

"Is everyone OK with 55 and 75?" asked the meeting chair. For some reason, several people raised their hands.

"OK, then—"

"Wait," said the man next to me. "Why do we need minimums for both parts?"

Several seconds of silence greeted that question.

"Good question," answered the chair. "You've got us thinking here."

Yeah, with MY question.

A few people chuckled at the chair's remark. The guy across the table from me said, "I think I'd rather have minimums so we know what our standards are."

That doesn't even make any sense.

However, most of the committee members were nodding their heads in agreement.

This is insane! Nobody in this room knows what the test measures or whether the communication part really does serve us better than computation.

And now we're actually thinking about just arbitrarily deciding that the 55-75 candidate is better qualified than the 54-99 one? Or the 100-74 one? How could we possibly know that?

"Any more discussion or should we vote on the minimums?" asked the chair.

If I raised my hand, I would have to talk. A lot. That means there would be many difficult words to struggle through. After all, there was much to say about the proposed plan.

Should I speak?

Let me first consider this from the other side. Devil's advocate and all that.

Would a 55-75 candidate really be so bad?

I mean, who's to say?

Questions:

Have you ever been afraid to speak up, even when you were clearly the smartest person in the room? Describe the situation, including any regrets you have.

Assuming the narrator would have stuttered when he spoke, how should he have handled the situation?

At the end of the story, he rationalizes that there is no way of knowing whether his ideas are really better. Why do you think he does that?

What if the narrator had spoken up and failed to convince the rest of the committee of the wrongness of their ideas—would he have wished he had kept quiet or would speaking up still have been better? Explain.

Were there any long-term costs to keeping quiet, or were they confined to that particular situation? Explain.

The committee was discussing ideas that seemed illogical and superficial to the narrator. Explain why you think the urge to remain quiet seemed to be as strong, if not stronger, than the urge to point out the craziness of what was being said.

Chapter 8: Stereotyped

I next found myself at a party. I was talking to a couple who seemed interested in the fact that I had attended a convention for people who stutter.

"I knew someone who stuttered once," said the woman. "Quiet guy. Understandably."

"Is that true of all people who stutter?" asked the man.

"Well, it's interesting—" I began.

"I'm sure it is," interrupted the woman. "After all, the person with a cane will limit how much he walks."

"That's not exactly the same—"

"But on the other hand," she continued, "it might help to practice speaking."

"Actually—"

"If I stuttered, I think I would practice until I got it right."

"It's not that sim—"

"I agree," said the man. "Practice makes perfect, as my old coach used to say."

With that, they both turned to me.

"You're pretty quiet too," said the woman.

I started to protest, but before I could say a word, another memory blast whisked me into a college pub. I was seated at the bar with my friend Tommy, but it was the stranger on the other side of me who had my attention.

"UT will win because they get better recruits," he said.

"That hasn't helped them much the puh-puh-puh…puh-puh-past couple of years," I noted.

"You don't know anything. State sucks."

I laughed. How is that even an argument?

Turning to Tommy, I said, "You about ready to go?"

"Yeah, you better look away," said the loudmouth UT fan. "Look away and hope I don't make you stand up for yourself."

I turned back toward him.

"What did you just say?"

But he was gone, replaced by my companion, looking like just another a derelict downing shots and beer.

"Did you look away because you were scared?"

"Honestly, that never crossed my mind," I said.

"I only looked elsewhere because that guh-guh-guh-guy seemed too stupid to carry on a decent conversation."

What I saw next was a well-dressed teen with slicked back hair and wire rimmed glasses. He was standing behind a podium. I was a high schooler again and he was my debating opponent.

"L-l-l-ladies and gentlemen, esteemed judges," he was saying, "my a-a-ad-ad-adversary is now granted a thirty second response."

Wow, I thought. This is great! Debates always made me nervous, but on this occasion, I was relaxed as I walked to the podium. Luck was with me. My opponent stuttered. He might be smart, but at least he would not be aggressive or mean.

"The puh-puh-problem," I began, "is that the same puh-pe-people who vote against tax increases for schools are the ones who complain about the quah-quality of those same schools. You can't have it both ways. If you are unwilling to pay for a puh-pruh-product, do not whine when said product is inferior."

I sat. My opponent rose and walked to his lectern. Then he spread his arms in an exaggerated gesture of confusion.

"I hardly know w-w-w-where to begin! F-f-first of all, the nay voters are not whining! They're merely exercising their right to vote as they see fit. M-m-m-m-more importantly, is it not possible that many of them have voted for such tax increases in the past, after which the money improved the schools not one iota?"

Hmm…I hadn't thought of that.

"A-a-a-and is it not also possible," he continued, "that they will vote for increases again, but only when they see a plan that shows them the money will be spent wisely?"

Several people in the crowd cheered at that.

Perhaps I had underestimated this guy.

Questions:

People who stutter are often stereotyped as shy, quiet, reserved, and introverted. How might that stereotype have impacted the conversation with the couple at the party?

_____

_____

_____

_____

_____

_____

Write out a self-fulfilling prophecy scenario from your own life (i.e., a situation in which you were induced to behave in a manner consistent with others' perceptions of you).

_____

_____

_____

_____

_____

_____

_____

_____

What would you change about the way you handled the situation?

_____

_____

_____

_____

_____

_____

_____

_____

Have you ever been stereotyped as quiet? Timid? Afraid? Have you ever felt like a magnet for bullies? Write your experience(s).

_____

_____

_____

_____

_____

_____

Have ever corrected someone who assumed you were quiet or timid (or any other false stereotype)? How did the other person react to being corrected? Would you handle the situation the same way again or would you change something?

_____

_____

_____

_____

_____

_____

_____

What other characteristics have been ascribed to you because of stuttering?

_____

_____

_____

_____

_____

_____

_____

Have you ever stereotyped someone else who stuttered? If yes, describe. If no, can you envision a scenario in which you might? Why would people who stutter stereotype each other, given that they know better?

Have you ever stereotyped anyone on a basis other than stuttering? Compare the experiences of being stereotyped vs. doing the stereotyping.

Chapter 9: Listeners

I. The Know-It-All

I found myself inside a convention center, so I must have been at a professional conference of some sort. I was holding a sandwich and drink, walking toward an empty table.

When I was seated and had taken my first bite, a man asked if he could join me. That sort of request is not uncommon at conferences, as the lunch tables are often large enough to seat eight or more and many attendees are there alone.

I nodded.

The man sat and immediately began speaking. "I liked your presentation today," he began.

"Thanks."

Then he got to what was on his mind. "I couldn't help but notice that you stutter."

I did not respond.

"I stuttered as a kid," he continued. "My dad told me he'd buy me a new bike if I stopped. Never stuttered again."

"Guh-guh-gruh-reat."

"Mind over matter, you know?"

I sighed.

"What?" he asked.

"That's not the way it works."

He laughed. "Who's the cured one here?"

"Look," I said, "I'm happy for you and all, but it's a complex disorder with no easy solution. I can't just decide to stop. We're not tuh-tuh-alking about belching in public here."

"I'm not saying it's simple. But you can summon your inner strength! When it comes right down to it, after all, it's just speech. Breathe, move your mouth, voila!"

"Speech is actually a very complicated process."

"But easy for humans to do."

"But duh-dih-disorders are hard to reverse. That's why stuttering has no cure."

He rolled his eyes. "Then explain why I don't stutter anymore." With that, he gave me his best mic drop look. I started to answer, but the scene before me changed.

II. The Jerk

The convention center transformed into a highway and the table to a car. I was jammed into the backseat with two friends from college. Two strangers sat in front. We were on our way back to campus from a football game. The car was packed full and I could not see my companion, though I again sensed it was close.

The stranger in the passenger seat turned to look at me. "Tell me," he said, "when you throw up, does the puke get stuck on its way out?"

This brought a laugh from the others in the car.

"Cruel," said one of my friends.

Emboldened, the stranger turned again, this time asking, "You ever consider becoming an auctioneer?"

The driver pretended like he was unsuccessfully suppressing laughter. "Ask him his name," he said. "That's always good for a laugh."

"OK. Hey, what's your name?"

I simply shook my head in response.

The stranger put his hand to his ear. "Whuh-whuh-whuh-whuh-what?"

He laughed hard at his own joke, then continued with, "I got a million of 'em."

As my new acquaintance entertained his audience, I contemplated my situation. Stuck in a car, my choices were few:

- Laugh along, after which I would hate myself;
- Don't laugh and look like a bad sport;
- Inform him that being mocked is hurtful; or
- Get angry, which is what the stranger wants.

As I contemplated these options, the road noise dissipated.

III. The Curious

I was standing now, in the middle of what appeared to be a shopping mall. I ran into a woman I knew from work and we started talking. Her child tugged on my shirt.

I looked down at the boy.

"Why do you talk like that?" he asked.

"Um..."

"Joey, that's rude!" said my colleague.

"But Mom, he doesn't just say the words. He goes uh uh uh or something."

"That's enough, Joey." Turning to me red-faced, she added, "I'm so sorry."

"That's OK," I said, although I wasn't really sure it was.

Behind the boy I spotted my companion, looking essentially like any other shopper, albeit one of the uglier ones.

I glanced at the boy's mother, who was now nearer to me. When I looked closer, I saw that she was another woman and the two of us were not in a mall but, rather, an elevator. I knew the drill well enough by then to understand that the scene was changing to a different memory.

IV. The Hypocrites

The elevator stopped on the fourth floor and I knew to exit. I was on my way to a meeting and would be just a minute or two late.

I felt no particular nerves about where I was going. I would be with a group of people with whom I had interacted plenty of times. Sometimes co-workers get too focused on how I speak and miss what I am saying, but these colleagues were good listeners. One had even told me that he doesn't really hear the stutter anymore. Another confided that she used to think to think of me as the stuttering co-worker, but now I was just another associate.

As I made my way down the hall toward the conference room, I saw that the door was open. Voices carried into the hallway.

"Who called this meeting?" asked one of them.

Another familiar voice answered, "Here's a h-h-h-h-hint."

Laughter followed.

"Good thing we set aside a full hour."

More laughter.

"That's really not nice," said a new voice. But it was said with a chuckle.

I stopped in my tracks, unsure whether to enter.

"A hundred percent true," said the same voice, "but still not nice."

The laughing resumed.

I decided to enter the room, to see if they were capable of shame. When I did so, all were grinning, but only one looked at me. As we locked eyes, he morphed into Cecile, woman I met in college.

V. The Benevolent

I arrived in the old dining hall in time to hear her say, "I don't really have any prejudices."

"I thought everyone did," I heard myself reply, my mind still in the process of getting focused on this new situation.

"Not anyone with a brain. Stereotyping is something done by the weak-minded."

At that point in time, Cecile was a fellow student in two of my classes. We had come to the moment when she was about to get more interested in me.

"Anyway," I began, "I thih-thih-thih-think I will get the tuh-tue-tuna sandwich."

"You stutter?!"

Behind her I saw my companion, ugly as always and sporting an evil grin. I nodded at Cecile's question.

"I knew someone in high school who stuttered! It was awful how people let him struggle. I was the only one who ever helped him!"

"Helped him? How?"

"If I knew what he was trying to say, I would finish his sentence. I asked questions in class for him. I even offered to stick up for him if anyone mocked his stutter."

"Puh-puh-perhaps I should explain some things to you..."

"I want to be your friend because I know that you'll be kind. Plus, you're very intelligent. It would be my honor to help you stick up for yourself."

As I was mulling over why she assumed I was nice, smart, and weak, I suddenly found myself inside the house in which I had grown up.

VI. Family

I was once again at the family dinner table. Perhaps this was the same scene I had jumped into and out of earlier. After all, around the table were my parents, brother, and me, all seated in the same chairs. My companion was not there, at least not visibly.

"How's school?" asked my mom.

"Fine," I answered. My younger brother Aaron nodded in agreement.

"Anything interesting happen?"

"Larry got cuh-cuh-caw-caught cheating.

"Really? What happened?"

"The tuh-tee-teacher was handing out the tuh-tests and said no more talking. Larry asked me if I had an extra puh-puh-pencil and the teacher guh-guh-gruh-grabbed his test, crumpled it up, and threw it on the floor.

"So what happens now?" asked my Dad.

"I guh-guh-guess he gets a zero."

"His parents are going to be furious!" exclaimed Mom. "Do you think the teacher will give him another chance?"

"I don't know. He was puh-preh-pretty mad."

"Larry better do well on the next test," said Aaron.

I began to calculate in my head. "Even if he gets a hundred on his next two tests, his average will still be a D."

"Wait," said Aaron. "How does that work?"

"One hundred plus one hundred plus zero equals two hundred. Two hundred divided by three is 67. Sixty-seven is a D."

"Holy—"

"Aaron!" warned my mom.

I didn't get to hear whether my brother finished his statement, for that was the moment that the scene switched to my first apartment as an adult. I was there with a friend. My companion was also present, looking surprisingly good.

VII. Friends

My first attempt at self-disclosure was with the friend who was now before me. We first met when we were in our twenties, when I was really good at hiding my stuttering. Through word substitution, rephrasing, and simply not talking, I was certain I had hidden my secret from him and pretty much everyone else. We stayed close for a number of years, and he came to visit after I got a job in a new town.

"What's going on with you?" he asked the day he arrived.

"Let's see, work, therapy, softball."

He nodded.

"Therapy for stuttering," I clarified.

"Uh huh."

This was not the reaction I was expecting, but I pressed on. I was determined to right a wrong.

"I don't think I ever tuh-told you, but I stutter."

"Duh."

"You knew?"

"I don't think I ever told you, but I have two legs."

I wasn't sure whether to laugh or feel disappointed. I did not have to decide, however, as the atmosphere soon became smoky and loud.

VIII. The Date

I met her in a bar. The place was crowded, and the music was loud. We were able to carry on a conversation, though I often felt like I was yelling.

Despite the trying circumstances, we spoke of work, family, movies, music, and a host of other topics. My throat was getting sore, but the conditions made fluent speech easy for a change, which was fun. I wanted the conversation to continue, but her friends announced they were leaving, and she had to go along.

"Can I call you?" I asked. The loudness level rose at that moment so I made a writing gesture so she could understand me over the din.

She smiled, then yelled, "I was wondering when you'd get around to asking me!" She took a pen and paper out of her purse and clearly wrote down her telephone number. When she handed it to me, I placed it inside a wallet sleeve to make sure I would not lose it.

The following day, then, it would be my job to call her. The problem was that making telephone calls had always been difficult for me. Or perhaps the real problem was that, if I called, she would hear the real me—stutter and all—for the first time.

I glanced across the bar and saw my companion, smiling in a way that was ugly, almost evil.

IX. The Subtle

I remained in the bar, or maybe it was a different one, I could not be sure. It seemed a bit quieter, so my speech was going to be tested more.

My friends were on the other side of the main seating area, so I sat at a table with friends of friends—people I had come with, but knew only marginally.

"How are you guh-guh-guys doing?" I asked as I took a seat.

The one nearest me produced what I took to be a condescending nod, then began conversing with the person to his left. After several exchanges, that individual looked at me.

"Waiting for tuh-tuh-tuh-Tom to get back?" I asked, referring to my friend across the room. I chuckled. "Once he starts socializing, there's no telling when he'll stop."

"Uh huh," was the response. Then the two of them resumed their conversation. Apparently, it got more amusing, as they began laughing.

After a few minutes, Tom returned.

"Buh-buh-'bout time you made it back," I said, happy to have someone to talk to.

But Tom looked at the others and asked, "What are you two laughing about?"

At that point, the three of them talked about whatever was so funny. I never found out what that was, as I had trouble hearing them from the other side of the table.

Questions:

Choose two people from among the know-it-alls, jerks, curious, hypocrites, etc. in your past and write your experiences.

Why did you choose the people you did?

If you could go back, what would you change about those situations?

How, in your opinion, should the narrator have handled the know-it-all?

How about the jerks in the car?

Children can be curious about stuttering. Is that suitable or rude? Explain your answer.

What would be the best response to a curious child?

What would you do if you overheard trusted allies making fun of you?
What should you do?

A co-worker claims to view the narrator as "just another colleague," yet makes fun of his stuttering behind his back. Can both of those things be true? Explain.

How do you feel about listeners who go to extremes to show they accept stuttering? It seems like a positive reaction, yet the narrator did not seem impressed. Why do you think that was?

The narrator again stuttered more when speaking to his parents, but not his brother. Speculate on why that might be the case.

He seemed disappointed that his friend already knew about his stuttering. Explain the disappointment. What role does the traveling companion play in that scene?

What should he do about the woman he met in the bar? Call and just be himself? Immediately self-disclose his stutter? What do you think you would do?

List 2 or 3 reasons why the friends of friends might have ignored the narrator in the bar.

Do you believe the actual reason had something to do with his stuttering? Explain.

Subtle prejudice does exist. People who do not even realize their own bias undoubtedly deny stuttering individuals everything from simple acknowledgement to promotions. Do you believe subtle prejudice has ever happened to you (e.g., you were ignored or overlooked for no apparent reason other than stuttering)? Describe an instance in which you believe this occurred to you.

Has subtle prejudice happened to you for reasons other than stuttering? If so, describe that instance.

Subtle prejudice can always be attributed to another reason. For example, the friends of friends, if challenged, might claim they were just continuing a previous conversation. Given how difficult it is to identify, can anything be done to combat it?

What do you wish listeners knew about stuttering? What do you wish they knew about your stuttering?

_____

_____

_____

_____

_____

_____

_____

Design your perfect listener. How realistic is your creation, i.e., does such a person exist?

_____

_____

_____

_____

_____

_____

_____

Chapter 10: Treatment

The next face I saw was that of my first speech-language pathologist. Unfortunately for me, she practiced in an era when continuing education was not mandatory for health professionals.

I was not so much having a conversation with her as I was listening to various proclamations, she had made during the school year when I met with her twice a week. That is, her image would tell me something and, before I could answer, it would disappear and reappear with a new declaration.

"Anyone can be fluent if they try hard enough," she announced on what must have been a cold day, given that she was wearing a wool sweater.

"We need to get at whatever the underlying issue is that's making you stutter. Tell me about your life." For that session, she wore a pantsuit and checkered blouse.

"If you talk slowly with a lot of air support, you can't stutter. It's simply impossible." Red dress for this one. Also, her hair was shorter and her face tanned.

"You can hit your targets with me. Just do the same thing everywhere else." The same red dress, oddly.

She faded away again. I assumed she would soon appear to impart more of her alleged wisdom, but instead I saw the face of my last SLP, making a new set of claims.

"You need to take responsibility for your own progress."

"There is no cure."

"There is no easy fix."

"You can't just learn techniques and, when you're ready, move them to all speaking situations. It doesn't work like that."

"Get outside of your comfort zone."

"The best way to learn how to deal with listener reactions to stuttering is to stutter with real listeners."

Questions:

Describe the differences between the two therapists in this chapter.

_____

_____

_____

_____

_____

_____

_____

_____

_____

_____

_____

_____

_____

Describe your best and worst therapy experiences. What would you change about your own behavior if you could relive them?

_____

_____

_____

_____

_____

_____

_____

_____

_____

_____

Pick 5 lessons learned from chapters 1-9. Relate them to therapy in some way. For example,

- Describe how they were taught to you in therapy
- Or note how they could be taught
- Or how they could have improved the treatment you received
- Or any other association you can make.

"Good treatment is more than just speech drills." Explain why you agree or disagree with this statement.

All told, the second therapist seems to be recommending getting out there and talking to people, with both fluent and stuttered speech. Is that good advice? Why or why not?

That same therapist mentions both learning new techniques and improving attitudes about speech. What do you think a good balance is between those two goals?

Chapter 11: Feeling Better About Stuttering

Old speech-language pathologists finally left me alone. Instead, I was on my office phone, explaining a company insurance policy to a new employee. My companion sat in the corner, looking presentable if not exactly attractive.

"I need more time to think about this," said the recent hire. "What if I sign up for the wrong benefit? Can I get out of it?"

"Duh-don't worry. I'm going to hold a meeting of all the new people and explain it in detail. That should help you duh-dud-dud-decide."

"Wait a minute, do you stutter?"

My face flushed. "Yes."

"And you're not afraid to present at a meeting? That's so cool! I don't stutter and public speaking scares me to death."

I was trying to decide whether thanking him was appropriate under the circumstances, but then I experienced another abrupt change of scenery, I found myself in support group meeting. Four regular attendees were there, plus my companion, who was all cleaned up for once. A long-time participant was talking.

"Where I work, stuttering would be devastating. If the higher-ups spot a weakness, they'll write you off in no time!"

"And stuttering's a weakness?" I asked.

"You bet it is. They wwwwwwant people who make a confident first impression, people who can talk to anybody."

"You can talk with cuh-cuh-confidence, even if you stutter."

"Easy for you to say. You're a mmmmmanager. People have to listen to you."

"Duh-do-do you think that was always the case? I wasn't born a manager."

"Hmm... OK, maybe not. So tell me how you got there."

"Same way anybody gets anywhere. A step at a time. Guh-guh-geh-get over one barrier, then another."

He considered my comment. "OK, I can rrrr-respect that," he said. "You've made the same journey, after all."

I was given no time to consider his words. I was next taken back to college, where I was outside, walking between the liberal arts building and my dormitory. A student in a motorized wheelchair was to my right, moving at about the same speed I was. I looked at him. He verbalized a quick greeting even though talking was clearly a strain for him. I walked a few steps further, then turned toward him again.

"Nice night," I commented.

His response sounded like "wuhh-a-wuhh-wuhh." He obviously had some difficulty with speech motor control.

I stopped and looked at him. He stopped too.

"I'm sorry, I didn't cuh-cuh-catch what you said."

He smiled. "Ahh wuhh juhh agee-en wih you."

I got that one. It would have been demeaning to congratulate him on getting his message across, so I just extended the conversation.

"Agreeing with me, eh? So you like it a little cool too?"

"Yaah."

"Where are you coming from?"

"Meeyee."

"Sorry. Missed it again."

"Meeyeeng!"

"Meeting?"

"Yaah."

"For what?"

"Skoo papuh."

That interested me. "You work for the school puh-puh-pay-paper?"

"Yaah."

"I thought about doing that. But then I somehow missed the first meeting."

"Ahh intoh-doo you."

"To who?"

"Hoom."

"Huh?"

He took a deep breath and repeated. "Ta whom."

"Fine, smart guy. To whom?"

He smiled at that. "Eh-uh-duh."

"The editor?"

He nodded, still smiling.

"That'd be cool. Thanks."

"He was true to his word too, introducing you to the newspaper's editor that very night. You and your new friend worked together on the campus newspaper for the next two years."

I looked to my left. Of course, the college student had been replaced by my traveling companion. Oddly, we were still walking across a campus stuck decades in the past. But I was no longer a twenty-year-old kid. Similarly, my companion looked like just another individual out for a walk.

"I learned something about myself that day," I said.

"That there are things worse than me?" It was said with a wink, as if knowing the suggestion was false.

I sighed. "No. The truth is 'it could be worse' argument doesn't work here. He turned out to be a better reporter, writer, and student than I was. I usually felt like the inferior one."

"So what was it you learned?"

I thought about it. "Any pride I take in befriending him has nothing to do with comparing our respective differences. I do, however, believe the lesson learned is about stuttering."

"See? I am good for something."

Questions:

List any positives you can think of about stuttering.

Are these 3 situations in this chapter positive in the same way? Explain.

Write about a positive situation of yours that involved stuttering.

Why did the narrator's face flush when he admitted to a new subordinate that he stuttered?

Overall, is stuttering a weakness, as suggested by the support group participant? Explain your answer.

Do some people perceive it to be a weakness, even if it's not?

What strengths does the narrator show in these situations? Write about a time you tapped into your strength(s) and achieved success. Include why you chose that particular story.

_____

_____

_____

_____

_____

_____

Has anyone ever benefitted from your experience as a person who stutters? Describe the situation(s).

_____

_____

_____

_____

_____

_____

_____

_____

Why do you think the student coming from the school newspaper meeting seemed to take a liking to the narrator?

_____

_____

_____

_____

_____

_____

At first glance, that story might, as the narrator noted, appear to be about stuttering comparing favorably to another condition. But the author is clear that it is not. What, then, did the narrator learn from that scenario?

What do you think he means by "…'it could be worse' doesn't work here"?

Chapter 12: Risk-taking

While I was contemplating matters related to my college newspaper, my age dropped four years and my surroundings became green and warm. I was on a soccer field. Twenty yards away stood my neighbor Horst.

I was never much of a soccer player, but working with Horst provided me an opportunity to improve. My twenty-something neighbor grew up playing the game in Germany and knew how to bend kicks. Even better, he said he would teach me. As I understood it, the keys were where my foot struck the ball and how I balanced my weight.

"Go," said Horst.

I set the ball in the corner of the field, backed up two steps, and gave it a ride. It bent around the cone Horst had placed a few feet from where he stood.

"Again," he commanded.

The cone was moved, but I still curved my kick around it.

"Again."

No problem. In the empty lot where we practiced, I could bend shots around cones, chairs, and whatever else Horst placed on the field.

I set the ball down and got ready to kick again. Only now there was no object on the field, just opposing players. The scene had changed subtly. It was probably mere months, perhaps even hours, past the neighborhood practice I had just left behind. I had some inkling of the game situation and my task was clear.

It was time to try my new skill in an actual game.

My school team played matches about once a week. It was a lax group, run by a phys ed teacher who wanted to coach football but had to settle for my teammates and me.

"Kick it!" he instructed me, as if I had anything else planned.

I approached the ball but suddenly the idea of curving it seemed impossible. Striking the ball in the exact right spot with my weight balanced correctly was, for reasons unknown, now a far-fetched idea.

"Kick it!"

I tried to remember all of Horst's instructions as I swung my foot. The ball curved not one iota and landed 30 feet out of bounds.

Both the opponents and my teammates started laughing.

"Such precision," mocked the goalie.

The referee, however, was waving his hands. He retrieved the ball and threw it back onto the field.

"No kick!" he yelled, then turned to me and said, "Wait for the whistle this time."

"You going to let him kick again?" a teammate yelled at my coach.

"Whatever," was the response.

I reset the ball. It would be easy to kick it straight in the general direction of the goal. No laughing, no mocking, and the game would continue like normal.

On the other hand, I had an opportunity to practice and perfect a new skill where I most wanted to use it.

"Kick it!"

I made up my mind and approached the ball. I swung my leg back, but it did not move.

The reason for my immobility, I suddenly realized, was that I was now seated in a diner. I had apparently ordered that most American of meals, a cheeseburger and fries, and was just noticing there was no ketchup on the table. I looked across the booth. There sat my companion, smiling and eating plain fries.

If I wanted ketchup, I would have to ask for it. The problem was that the word in question had always been one of my most feared.

My choices were to 1) stutter openly, 2) attempt to modify my fluency by taking a deep breath and easing into the word, 3) modify the stutter with an easy bounce of k-k-k-k-ketchup, or 4) use a controlled stutter on another word in the sentence. Of course, there was a fifth option—shut up and not deal with stuttering in any fashion. That was the easiest solution, but I decided that my companion was not going to win this round.

I motioned the server over to the table.

"May I help you?" she asked.

Yes, I thought. You can help me execute option 4.

"I wwwwwwould like sssssome ketchup please."

She quickly grabbed a bottle from a nearby table and set it in front of me.

"Anything else?" she asked with a smile.

I shook my head. The ketchup and the moment were enough for now.

I next found myself in a high school parking lot, directing cars to open spaces. I had been roped into volunteering for this all-day task by my friend Lars, whose daughter was a freshman at the school.

The event was a marching band competition that would be well attended.

I was there because not enough parents had volunteered and thus the parking crew was shorthanded. Moreover, none of the six of us, including me, had any idea what we were doing when the day began. Through trial and error, however, we had developed a system whereby we motioned cars into the main entrance, then to the lots with open spaces. It was efficient and gave the attendees some options where to park.

The school's principal came out of his office and called the parking volunteers over to where he stood.

"You want to fill in the spaces one at a time," he said, "starting with ones furthest from school."

"Why furthest?" asked Lars.

"To keep cars away from pedestrians."

I didn't want to speak, but could sense annoyance among my cohorts. What the heck, I thought, I don't have a child in the school.

"Actually, our way is working juh-juh-juh-just fine. Let's not fix what isn't buh-bruh-broken."

The principal glanced at me, then looked at the others. Something in their faces made him want to defend himself.

"It's not orderly."

"So what—?" I began.

"I don't have time to explain it to you. Just do as I say." With that, he walked back toward the school's entrance.

It was now or never.

"Hey!" My exclamation came out louder than I had planned, but so be it. All six of the men gathered looked at me.

"Duh-duh-don't walk away in the middle of the conversation. I wasn't finished."

The principal stopped and slowly turned.

"OK," he finally said.

"There is absolutely no reason to change the system. The puh-puh-puh-peh-pedestrians are on the sidewalks, so there is no safety issue. Let puh-puh-people park where they want."

The principal simply nodded, then went back into the building.

"Thanks," whispered Lars.

Questions:

What do the 3 stories in this chapter have in common?

_____

_____

_____

_____

_____

_____

_____

What does the soccer story have to do with stuttering?

_____

_____

_____

_____

_____

_____

Describe a situation in which you had to make a choice between taking a risk and playing it safe.

_____

_____

_____

_____

_____

_____

_____

Describe a situation (speech or otherwise) in which you took a risk (use the one from the previous question if you wish). Why did you take the chance you did? How did you feel during the risk and after?

Describe a situation (speech or otherwise) in which you chickened out. Explain why you opted out and how you felt afterward.

What do you believe the narrator would have done had he been able to kick the ball a second time—try to bend it or just put it in play? Explain your answer.

When he was in the diner, why didn't he just eat his fries plain?

What do you think changed from the meeting in chapter 7 to the diner scene?

He yelled at the school's principal louder than he intended to, then quickly brushed off this unsociable action. Why did it not concern him?

If you didn't already do so above, describe a situation in which you took a risk with your stuttering.

Do you believe taking risks outside of stuttering can help one to lead a more meaningful life? Explain your answer.

List examples of when 1) you took a risk and it paid off and 2) you took a risk and failed. What did you learn from these experiences?

Repeat the previous exercise with speech risks.

Can risks gone wrong still be valuable experiences? Why or why not?

Chapter 13: Acceptance

"So," began Lars (my friend who had roped me into parking duty), "what's the deal with your speech?"

"I stutter."

"That much I figured out. Why?"

"Don't know."

"How do you make it stop?"

"Don't know."

"So what do you do about it?"

"Just talk."

"And stutter?"

"Sometimes."

"And you don't care?"

That question gave me pause. "It's not that I don't care exactly," I finally said. "It's still inconvenient and I'd rather not do it. I guess like everyone else, I just play the cards life dealt me."

"Let's get to our seats," answered Lars. In context, this command made no sense. I looked at him and realized that I was now talking to a neighbor of mine. We had gone to a football game together and were making our way through the stadium.

I also noticed that we were both dressed in solid red, as were most of the other people shuffling toward the upper deck. The rest were in green.

About then, two of the green fans passed by. The taller of them yelled, "Get ready to be owned, wee ones!"

"Puh-puh-puh-pure genius," I said to my neighbor. He laughed.

Unbeknownst to me, the tall green guy was watching me as I spoke. Within seconds, he was directly in front of me.

"Whuh-whuh-what did you say?" he said, laughing for the benefit of his cohort. "Taw-taw-talk much?"

My neighbor and I kept walking. After a few seconds, he said, "I hope that's not a sign of the kinds of idiots we have to deal with tonight."

"You know," I said, considering the situation, "stuttering is easy to make fun of. Stupid tuh-tuh-takes more effort."

We both laughed.

Then I was no longer in a football stadium. There were sheets on me and a pillow beneath my head. I looked at the clock radio. It read 5:25 am.

Almost time to get up. I decided to wait for the alarm, to take the five minutes of rest

I had coming to me.

I sensed my companion was near and I was correct. I can't say with any sort of accuracy how long it took the image to come into view, but it wasn't immediate. Nor was it worth the wait.

Most would have found it forgettable, perhaps even homely, but I was used to it in all its forms.

The formation knew me on sight, of course, and made its presence known. However, I had other things to think about. There was road construction on the nearby highway, so I would have to leave the house a little early. The day was full: meetings and clients and a phone conference to end the afternoon. Hopefully, that would not last long, as I needed to make a quick trip to the grocery store on the way home. The car was low on gas too, so I had to figure that stop in as well.

A giant arm gestured for me to follow. I viewed that only as a request, one I could ignore.

Maybe I can drive city streets in to work today, I thought. That way, I could avoid the highway construction and get gas in the morning instead of after 5 when the stations were all crowded.

The image danced around, trying desperately to get my attention. I shook my head.

Keep dancing, tough guy.

There's no power in dancing. The alarm buzzed and I got out of bed.

Time to start a new day.

Questions:

Given that there is no cure for stuttering, how can it best be managed?

The narrator defines acceptance as, "It's not that I don't care exactly. It's still inconvenient and I'd rather not do it. I guess like everyone else, I just play the cards life dealt me." Is that a reasonable way to look at it? What is your definition?

This chapter follows one on risk-taking. How is that concept related to acceptance?

Do you believe you have accepted your stuttering? Why or why not?

In what other areas of life have you gained acceptance? How do those self-approvals differ from accepting stuttering?

What indicators show you (or would show you) that you are becoming more accepting of your speech?

Did the narrator and his neighbor handle the obnoxious fan appropriately? Why or why not? What would you have done?

At the end of the chapter, the companion is, for the first time, ignored. Why?

Compare the final scene to the opening of chapter 1. How are they similar? How are they different? Why are they different?

Is the "new day" he is about to start (in the last line of the chapter) going to be just another day? Explain your answer.

_____

_____

_____

_____

_____

_____

"There's no power in dancing," he says. Is there power in acceptance? Why or why not?

_____

_____

_____

_____

_____

_____

_____

Final Questions

No matter how well someone confronts it, accepts it, and moves past it, sometimes the companion is successful at becoming an interference again. What can be done in those instances? In other words, how best can its power be diminished again?

Different things work for different people. Below are some ideas from this workbook. Write down the pros and cons of each, focusing on how well you believe they would help you regain power over it.

- Open stuttering, without avoidance, fear, or embarrassment
- Voluntary stuttering on words you could have said fluently
- Self-disclose your stuttering
- Openly use techniques you learned in therapy
- Say feared words knowing you will stutter
- Speak (and stutter) in feared situations
- Use humor
- Go through this workbook again
- Return to (or begin) therapy
- Read the following essays about relapse:
    ◊ Fraser, M. Self-Therapy for the Stutterer. Excerpted at: https://www. stutteringhelp.org/do-you-get-discouraged
    ◊ Pollard, R. Relapse Following Successful Stuttering Therapy. The Problem of Choice. Available at: https://www.mnsu.edu/comdis/isad16/papers/pollard16. html
    ◊ Starkweather, C.W. Relapse: A Misnomer. Available at: https://www.stuttering-specialist.com/post/relapse-a-misnomer
- Other ideas (please specify)

Go out and use the ideas listed above. Try them separately and in combinations. How well does each strategy keep you on track (or put you back on track) toward managing your stutter? Look at the ones that work for you. Why do you think they are successful?

Appendix: Where to go from here

If there existed a stuttering bookstore, it would be like all other such shops: filled with a variety of customers, all looking for different items. Some would want books on speech techniques, others on dealing with emotions. There would be those searching for the self-help section and probably a large group there simply to browse.

Given that I don't know what sort(s) of information you have your eye on, this chapter will include on-line stuttering resources that cover all sections of the imaginary bookstore. It is not an exhaustive list, but hopefully it can help some of you find what you are looking for.

Treatment

We can begin with therapy. Resources that are valuable in the search for a speech-language pathologist (SLP) proficient in the treatment of stuttering include:

- Australian Speak Easy Association
    - ◊ Speak Easy provides links to resources that can help those in need find an SLP near them.
- The Canadian Stuttering Association
    - ◊ There are tabs to help find an SLP in any area of the country.
- International Fluency Association
    - ◊ The About Us link brings the reader to a drop-down menu with "IFA Experts" and their respective locations around the world.
- Speech Pathology Australia
    - ◊ This site offers multiple sources for stuttering therapy in Australia. One of the most helpful pages is "Find a SLP" which matches therapists to geographic information.
- Stuttering Foundation (America)
    - ◊ The Stuttering Foundation website has a tab for referrals for speech-language pathologists with an interest in treating stuttering.
- Stuttering Foundation (Australia)
    - ◊ This site has a link for SLP referrals in Australia.
- Stutteringspecialist.org
    - ◊ This is the website for the American Board of Fluency and Fluency Disorders (ABFFD).
    - ◊ ABFFD board-certified specialists in fluency (BCS-F) across the US are listed.

Support

- Australian Speak Easy Association
  - ◊ In addition to treatment help, readers can connect to support groups throughout Australia.
- Brazilian Stuttering Association
  - ◊ This site includes links to support groups for parents and people who stutter in Brazil.
- British Stammering Association
  - ◊ BSA provides information about self-help groups (on-line and in-person) and presentations about stuttering.
- The Canadian Stuttering Association
  - ◊ CSA links supply material about support groups in all areas of Canada.
- Facebook
  - ◊ Facebook includes numerous pages dedicated to support, including the following.
    - Stuttering Community
    - Stuttering Hangout
    - Stuttering Arena
    - NSA Chapter Pages
    - Stutter School
- Friends
  - ◊ Friends has their own mentoring program for children who stutter, by teens who stutter.
  - ◊ There are also links for their annual convention and one-day conferences.
- National Stuttering Association (NSA)
  - ◊ The website provides information about NSA local chapters across the US. This includes Teens Who Stutter (TWST) groups.
  - ◊ The NSA has an annual conference in which professionals and people who stutter present research and advice about various aspects of the disorder. It is also a place for people who stutter to get together informally to share and listen to others' experiences.
- Stuttering Answers
  - ◊ Stuttering Answers offers information about stuttering and stuttering support groups. There is an easily accessible tab which provides the times and places of support group meetings across Australia.

- Stuttering Association for the Young (SAY)
  - ◊ Camp SAY is a sleep-away summer camp to empower young people who stutter and help them build connections in the stuttering community.
- Stuttersocial.com
  - ◊ This website provides access to group video chats for people who stutter. It is a safe place for people to make friends and share experiences with other people who stutter.

Resources

- American Speech Hearing Association (ASHA)
  - ◊ The ASHA website provides general information about stuttering as well as links to resources for people who stutter.
- Brazilian Stuttering Association
  - ◊ This site offers multiple resources for people who stutter.
- British Stammering Association
  - ◊ This website provides links for stuttering information for different age groups.
- The Canadian Stuttering Association
  - ◊ Resources in North America and Europe are listed.
- Friends
  - ◊ The website includes information about stuttering for parents, teens, and children.
  - ◊ Their Stuttering 101 tab provides basic information about stuttering.
- The International Fluency Association
  - ◊ The Links tab on this website delivers readers to multiple resources for people who stutter all over the world.
  - ◊ The News link brings them to a variety of stuttering-related news articles.
- International Stuttering Association
  - ◊ A resources tab connects to a list of stuttering-related materials for children, teachers, and parents.
- Make Room for the Stuttering - StutterRockstar.com
  - ◊ This is primarily a blog, founded by a woman who stutters and geared primarily toward women who stutter. It includes posts and podcasts on a variety of topics.
- National Stuttering Association (NSA)
  - ◊ The NSA website has a multitude of resources that cover almost every aspect of stuttering. They also provide information about research and other news about the disorder.
- Stuttering Foundation
  - ◊ There is a tab for resources that will bring the user to brochures, free e-books, and videos that deal with topics related to stuttering. There are also downloadable versions of all the foundation's past newsletters.
- Stuttering is Cool
  - ◊ This website contains podcasts on various topics related to stuttering.

- StutterTalk
  - ◊ This resource includes multiple podcasts on varying topics and from a wide variety of people.
- The Stuttering Source
  - ◊ This site includes a resources tab that links to other websites and blogs about stuttering.
  - ◊ There are also forms and brochures that are mainly for parents but can be useful for understanding stuttering.
- We Stutter @ Work
  - ◊ Webinar series focused on the workplace.
- YouTube
  - ◊ There is a variety of material on stuttering, ranging from Tedx Talks about the experience of stuttering to comedy channels, such as those of Jaik Campbell, Nina G, and Drew Lynch.

And finally,

- The Stuttering Homepage
  - ◊ If you don't find what you're looking for, don't give up without first checking out the SHP: https://www.mnsu.edu/comdis/kuster/stutter.html. There is a Therapy for Stuttering tab which includes information on various therapy techniques. Support group information and links are also available, as are general resources. Finally, if you seek information about countries other than those listed within this chapter, use the Stuttering in other Countries/Cultures tab.

www.ingramcontent.com/pod-product-compliance
Lightning Source LLC
Chambersburg PA
CBHW080253030426
42334CB00023BA/2799

9780987347657